The POTS Compass

Empowering Strategies, Insights, and Graceful Support for Postural Orthostatic Tachycardia Syndrome

Donna Stradley

Table of Contents

INTRODUCTION

In my journey as a medical professional specializing in the complexities of Postural Orthostatic Tachycardia Syndrome (POTS), I've been privileged to witness the resilience and courage of those battling this condition. POTS is more than a medical diagnosis; it's a life-altering experience that challenges every aspect of daily living, from physical endurance to emotional resilience. This book, "The POTS Compass," is born from a deep-seated desire to bridge the gap between clinical knowledge and the lived experience of those affected. It aims to be more than a medical guide; it seeks to be a beacon of understanding and support, illuminating a path through the often confusing and challenging landscape of POTS.

The heart of this book lies in its mission to empower. Whether you've recently been diagnosed, are a veteran in managing POTS, a caregiver seeking understanding, or a medical professional looking for deeper insights, this book is written for you. It is designed to unravel the complexities of POTS, demystifying symptoms, exploring the physiological mechanisms at play, and most importantly, providing practical strategies to manage life with this condition. This book goes beyond the scope of conventional medical texts, aiming to be a source of hope, inspiration, and actionable guidance.

I believe strongly in the power of knowledge, but even more in the power of shared experiences and community. This book is enriched with personal stories and case studies, offering a window into the lives of individuals with POTS. These stories are not just narratives; they are lifelines of shared experiences and collective wisdom. They provide comfort in knowing that while each journey with POTS is unique, there are common threads of challenge, resilience, and triumph.

As we delve into the present understanding of POTS, covering current treatment options, lifestyle adaptations, and coping strategies, we also look toward the future. This book delves into the latest research, emerging therapies, and the evolving landscape of POTS treatment. It's a commitment to staying abreast of advancements and innovations, providing you with the most current information and hope for future developments.

"The POTS Compass" is an invitation to a journey. This book stands as a steadfast companion, a guide through the uncertainties, and a source of solace and understanding. It's a commitment to walk with you through the complexities of POTS, facing challenges together, celebrating the victories, no matter how small, and empowering you to take an active role in managing your condition.

This book is also a conversation starter, aiming to bring POTS into the broader dialogue about chronic illness management and patient-centered care. It's an advocate for increased awareness and understanding, both in the medical community and the public sphere. By sharing knowledge, experiences, and insights, we can foster a more empathetic and informed approach to living with and treating POTS.

As you turn these pages, I invite you to engage with an open mind and heart. May this book serve as a source of knowledge, a beacon of hope, and a testament to the strength and resilience inherent in each person affected by POTS. Together, let us navigate the challenges and embrace the possibilities that lie ahead in your journey with POTS.

CHAPTER ONE: UNDERSTANDING POTS

This chapter is dedicated to thoroughly defining POTS, examining its diverse symptoms, and detailing the diagnostic process, while also addressing the issue of common misdiagnoses. We delve into the physiology behind POTS, shedding light on the malfunction of the autonomic nervous system that lies at the heart of this syndrome. Understanding the triggers and factors that can worsen POTS symptoms is crucial, and we provide insights into these elements for effective condition management.

Furthermore, we differentiate POTS from other similar medical conditions, emphasizing its unique features and how it stands apart from other disorders with similar symptoms or comorbidities. Aimed at patients, caregivers, and healthcare professionals, this chapter sets a solid foundation for the comprehensive understanding of POTS, its impacts, and its management.

Defining POTS: Symptoms and Diagnosis

Postural Orthostatic Tachycardia Syndrome (POTS) represents a multifaceted autonomic disorder characterized primarily by an excessive increase in heart rate upon standing. This condition is part of a group of disorders known as orthostatic intolerance. The cardinal symptom of POTS is a significant increase in heart rate –

typically 30 beats per minute (bpm) or more – within 10 minutes of assuming an upright position, without an accompanying drop in blood pressure. This symptom is a manifestation of the dysfunction in the autonomic nervous system, particularly the sympathetic nervous system, which is responsible for the body's 'fight-or-flight' responses.

In-Depth Look at Common Symptoms

Postural Orthostatic Tachycardia Syndrome (POTS) is a disorder characterized by a variety of symptoms, each contributing to the complexity and challenge of managing this condition. Understanding these symptoms in detail is crucial for both patients and healthcare providers to effectively navigate the intricacies of POTS.

Tachycardia: The most defining symptom of POTS is tachycardia, a rapid increase in heart rate upon standing. This increase typically exceeds 30 beats per minute (bpm) or a total heart rate that surpasses 120 bpm. Patients often experience palpitations, where they can feel their heart racing or pounding in their chest. This sensation can be distressing, causing anxiety and discomfort. Tachycardia in POTS is not just an isolated cardiac issue; it's a symptom of broader autonomic dysfunction.

Dizziness and Lightheadedness: Dizziness and lightheadedness in POTS are primarily due to orthostatic intolerance – the body's inability to adjust to an upright position. This leads to decreased cerebral blood flow when standing, causing symptoms that range from mild dizziness to severe lightheadedness and even fainting. These symptoms can significantly impair a person's ability to perform everyday tasks and can increase the risk of falls and injuries.

Chronic Fatigue: Chronic fatigue in POTS is profound and debilitating. Unlike normal tiredness, it doesn't improve with rest and can persist over long periods. This fatigue severely limits a person's physical and cognitive abilities, affecting their daily routines, work productivity, and overall quality of life. Patients often describe this fatigue as feeling drained or physically 'heavy', even after minor activities.

Heart Palpitations: Heart palpitations in POTS are sensations where the heartbeat feels abnormally strong, rapid, or irregular. They are not only physically uncomfortable but can also be psychologically distressing, as patients may worry about their heart health. These palpitations can be more noticeable during tachycardia episodes, after physical activity, or even during periods of rest.

Cognitive Dysfunction (Brain Fog): Cognitive dysfunction, often referred to as 'brain fog', is a common symptom in POTS. It includes difficulties with concentration, memory lapses, and a general sense of mental cloudiness. This can significantly impact personal and professional life, making tasks that require mental clarity and focus challenging. Patients may struggle with everyday cognitive demands, from remembering appointments to concentrating at work or school.

Headaches: Headaches in POTS patients can vary in type and severity. They range from mild tension headaches to severe migraines and are often exacerbated by physical activity, prolonged standing, or during periods of intense tachycardia. These headaches can further complicate the management of POTS, as they add another layer of discomfort and can be debilitating.

Gastrointestinal Disturbances: Gastrointestinal symptoms, including nausea, abdominal pain, bloating, constipation, and diarrhea, are frequently reported by POTS patients. These symptoms are believed to result from autonomic nervous system dysfunction affecting digestive processes. The variability and unpredictability of these symptoms can complicate dietary management and overall nutrition, impacting the patient's health and well-being.

Shaking and Sweating: Physical manifestations of the body's exaggerated sympathetic response, such as shaking and sweating, are common during episodes of increased heart rate in POTS. These symptoms can be uncomfortable and may cause social anxiety, complicating the patient's ability to engage in social interactions and professional activities.

Exercise Intolerance: Many individuals with POTS experience difficulty with physical exertion. Activities that increase heart rate can significantly exacerbate symptoms, particularly tachycardia and fatigue. This intolerance often leads to a decrease in overall fitness and physical health, creating a cycle that can worsen POTS symptoms over time.

Temperature Regulation Issues: POTS patients may exhibit intolerance to heat or cold, which can worsen their symptoms. This intolerance presents challenges in various environments, affecting comfort and limiting the ability to engage in outdoor activities or withstand certain workplace conditions.

Understanding these symptoms and their impact on everyday life is essential for effective management and treatment of POTS. Each symptom not only represents a physical challenge but also contributes to the emotional and psychological burden of living with this condition.

Criteria for Diagnosis

Diagnosing Postural Orthostatic Tachycardia Syndrome (POTS) is a multifaceted process that hinges on a combination of symptomatic presentation, patient history, and objective diagnostic criteria. Due to the overlap of POTS symptoms with other disorders and their variable presentation, a detailed and careful approach is essential for an accurate diagnosis. Here is an in-depth exploration of the criteria and processes involved in diagnosing POTS.

Key Diagnostic Criteria

The diagnosis of POTS is primarily based on the observation of specific cardiovascular responses to standing or upright posture. The widely accepted criteria include:

Heart Rate Increase: The most crucial criterion for POTS is a marked increase in heart rate upon standing. Specifically, this involves an increase of 30 beats per minute (bpm) or more within 10 minutes of standing or tilting up for adults, or 40 bpm or more for adolescents. This increase should occur in the absence of significant orthostatic hypotension (a drop in blood pressure of more than 20/10 mmHg).

Additional Diagnostic Considerations

In addition to the heart rate criteria, several other factors are considered essential for a comprehensive diagnosis:

Symptom Duration: Symptoms consistent with POTS should be present for at least six months. This duration helps distinguish POTS from transient conditions and ensures that the symptoms are chronic and sustained.

Exclusion of Other Causes: A thorough investigation to exclude other causes of the symptoms is a critical step. This includes ruling out conditions such as dehydration, medication side effects, prolonged bed rest, or other cardiovascular or autonomic disorders. Specific blood tests may be necessary to exclude conditions like anemia, hyperthyroidism, or pheochromocytoma.

Age of Onset: While POTS can occur at any age, it is most frequently diagnosed in adolescents and young adults, often following puberty or a significant illness or trauma. The age at which symptoms begin can provide valuable clues for diagnosis.

Diagnostic Tests

A series of tests are employed to confirm a POTS diagnosis and to rule out other potential causes of the symptoms:

Tilt Table Test: This test is the gold standard for POTS diagnosis. The patient is strapped to a table, which is then tilted to mimic the change from lying to standing. Heart rate and blood pressure are monitored throughout the test to observe the body's response to the change in posture.

Blood and Urine Tests: These tests can identify or rule out various conditions that might present with similar symptoms, such as metabolic disorders, endocrine abnormalities, or infections.

Echocardiogram: To exclude any underlying heart disease or structural abnormalities, an echocardiogram might be conducted to provide a detailed view of the heart's structure and function.

24-Hour Holter Monitor: This continuous recording of the heart's electrical activity can help detect any underlying rhythm abnormalities that might contribute to or complicate the clinical picture of POTS.

Assessing for Comorbid Conditions

POTS often doesn't occur in isolation. Recognizing and managing comorbid conditions such as Ehlers-Danlos Syndrome, Mast Cell Activation Syndrome, or Chronic Fatigue Syndrome is crucial. These conditions can exacerbate POTS symptoms and may influence both the diagnosis and management strategies.

Patient History and Physical Examination

A detailed patient history is indispensable in the diagnosis of POTS. The healthcare provider will inquire about the onset, duration, and pattern of symptoms, as well as any potential triggers or relieving factors. A comprehensive physical examination, including orthostatic vital signs, can provide additional clues to a POTS diagnosis. Documenting the patient's response to prolonged standing or changes in posture is particularly valuable.

The Role of Patient Observation and Reporting

Patients are often asked to keep a diary of their symptoms, noting their activities, meals, stress levels, and symptoms throughout the day. This diary can be invaluable in identifying patterns and triggers for POTS symptoms, assisting in both diagnosis and management.

Collaboration Among Specialists

Given the complex nature of POTS and its potential overlap with other disorders, a multidisciplinary team approach is often necessary. This team may include cardiologists, neurologists, and other specialists who can contribute to a comprehensive evaluation and diagnosis.

Diagnosing POTS is a careful balancing act that requires consideration of a wide array of symptoms, test results, and patient history. It's a process that not only involves identifying the presence of POTS but also differentiating it from other possible conditions. With a detailed and patient-centered approach, healthcare providers can accurately diagnose POTS, paving the way for effective management and improved quality of life for patients.

Navigating Common Misdiagnoses

The diagnostic journey for patients with Postural Orthostatic Tachycardia Syndrome (POTS) is often complex and riddled with potential misdiagnoses. The symptoms of POTS overlap significantly with various other medical conditions, leading to confusion and delays in receiving appropriate care.

Misdiagnosis as Anxiety or Panic Disorders: One of the most common misdiagnoses for POTS is anxiety or panic disorders. The palpitations, rapid heartbeat, and shortness of breath that are characteristic of POTS closely resemble the symptoms of anxiety attacks. Consequently, patients are sometimes mistakenly treated for anxiety, receiving therapies or medications that do not address the autonomic dysfunction central to POTS. This misdiagnosis can result in prolonged distress and ineffective treatment for the patient.

Confusion with Chronic Fatigue Syndrome (CFS): Chronic Fatigue Syndrome (CFS) and POTS share several symptoms, including debilitating fatigue, cognitive impairment (often referred to as 'brain fog'), and exercise intolerance. However, while both conditions involve significant fatigue, the presence of orthostatic intolerance – symptoms that worsen upon standing – is more indicative of POTS. Distinguishing between these two conditions is critical, as they require different management approaches.

Mistaking POTS for Orthostatic Hypotension: POTS is often confused with orthostatic hypotension, as both conditions involve symptoms upon standing, such as dizziness and lightheadedness. The key difference lies in the blood pressure response: orthostatic hypotension is characterized by a significant decrease in blood pressure upon standing, unlike POTS, which primarily involves an increase in heart rate. Accurate measurement of both heart rate and blood pressure upon standing is essential to differentiate between these conditions.

Misattribution to Dehydration or Poor Diet: Especially in younger patients, symptoms of POTS such as dizziness, fatigue, and increased heart rate are sometimes wrongly attributed to lifestyle factors like dehydration or poor diet. While these factors can exacerbate POTS symptoms, they are not the underlying cause. A thorough medical evaluation is necessary to identify the autonomic dysfunction characteristic of POTS and to differentiate it from these more benign causes.

Overlooking Other Autonomic Disorders: Other autonomic disorders, like neurally mediated hypotension or vasovagal syncope, can mimic POTS symptoms. These conditions also involve autonomic dysfunction but have different triggers and manifestations. Distinguishing POTS from these conditions requires detailed autonomic testing, including tilt table tests and careful observation of heart rate and blood pressure responses to various stimuli.

The Role of Patient Advocacy: Patients often play a critical role in navigating the diagnosis of POTS. Due to the condition's complexity and the potential for misdiagnosis, patient advocacy is essential.

Patients are encouraged to be proactive in discussing their symptoms in detail, seeking second opinions, and consulting with specialists who are familiar with POTS. Educating oneself about the distinct features of POTS can empower patients to advocate for appropriate testing and treatment.

In summary, accurately diagnosing POTS demands a careful and informed approach from both medical professionals and patients. Awareness of the condition's symptomatology and the potential for misdiagnosis is key to ensuring that patients receive the correct diagnosis and appropriate management for their symptoms.

Recognizing and accurately diagnosing POTS is a crucial step toward effective management and treatment. It requires a holistic understanding of the patient's symptoms, a thorough review of medical history, and often, collaboration among various healthcare professionals. This chapter aims to provide a detailed and nuanced understanding of the symptoms associated with POTS and the rigorous process involved in its diagnosis, thus laying the groundwork for exploring subsequent treatment and management strategies.

The Physiology Behind POTS

Understanding Postural Orthostatic Tachycardia Syndrome (POTS) requires an in-depth look at the autonomic nervous system (ANS) and its intricate workings, as the dysfunction of this system lies at the heart of the disorder. The ANS, a crucial part of the human body, regulates involuntary physiological processes like heart rate, blood pressure, digestion, and respiratory rate. It operates subconsciously and is divided into the sympathetic and parasympathetic nervous systems, each playing a vital role in maintaining bodily equilibrium.

The sympathetic system, often referred to as the 'fight or flight' system, prepares the body for stressful situations by increasing heart rate, raising blood pressure, and redirecting blood flow to essential organs. In contrast, the parasympathetic system, known as the 'rest and digest' system, conserves energy, reduces heart rate, and aids in digestion. In POTS, the balance between these two systems is disrupted, particularly in response to postural changes. Usually, when someone is standing up, gravity leads to blood accumulating in the lower parts of the body.

The ANS compensates for this by constricting blood vessels and slightly increasing the heart rate to maintain blood flow to the brain and vital organs. However, in POTS, this compensatory mechanism fails. There is often inadequate vasoconstriction in the lower body, leading to abnormal pooling of blood in the legs. In response, the body's heart rate increases excessively, an attempt to maintain cerebral perfusion, but this is not a fully effective response and leads to the hallmark symptom of POTS – an excessive increase in heart rate upon standing.

The exact mechanisms leading to ANS dysfunction in POTS are not entirely understood and are likely multifactorial. Theories include peripheral denervation, suggesting a partial neuropathy or damage to the nerves in the lower limbs that impairs their ability to signal for proper vasoconstriction. Another theory is the hyperadrenergic state in some POTS patients, where there is an excessive release of norepinephrine, a neurotransmitter of the sympathetic nervous system, causing an exaggerated response to standing.

Additionally, reduced blood volume or hypovolemia in POTS can exacerbate the pooling of blood in the legs and the compensatory tachycardia. For some individuals, POTS may have an autoimmune component, where the immune system mistakenly attacks components of the ANS. Genetic predisposition might also play a role, making certain individuals more likely to develop POTS.

In understanding the physiology of POTS, it is also crucial to consider that this condition is not uniform across all patients. The variability in symptoms and severity among individuals with POTS is reflective of the diverse ways in which the ANS can be affected. This complexity necessitates a personalized approach to treatment and underscores the importance of a nuanced understanding of the condition for both patients and healthcare providers. The varied and complex nature of ANS dysfunction in POTS makes it a challenging condition to manage effectively, requiring ongoing research and a comprehensive, patient-centric approach to care.

Common Triggers and Aggravating Factors

Understanding the triggers and aggravating factors of Postural Orthostatic Tachycardia Syndrome (POTS) is vital for those affected to manage their condition effectively. POTS is a multifaceted disorder, and various environmental, physiological, and lifestyle factors can exacerbate its symptoms. Recognizing these can help in crafting a personalized management plan to mitigate the impacts of these triggers.

Environmental Triggers

Heat Exposure: Heat induces vasodilation, increasing the tendency for blood to pool in the legs and exacerbating symptoms of orthostatic intolerance. Hot weather, hot showers, or environments like saunas can be particularly challenging, leading to increased fatigue, dizziness, and tachycardia.

Prolonged Standing or Upright Posture: Standing for long periods can increase orthostatic stress, leading to more pronounced blood pooling and subsequent tachycardia and fatigue. Jobs or situations requiring extended standing can significantly aggravate symptoms.

High Altitude: Changes in altitude affect oxygen levels and can strain the cardiovascular system, often leading to an increase in heart rate and exacerbating POTS symptoms. The lower air pressure at high altitudes can also affect blood volume regulation.

Dietary and Hydration Factors

Alcohol and Caffeine Consumption: Both substances can affect vascular tone and heart rate. Alcohol can lead to dehydration, exacerbating the hypovolemia often seen in POTS, while caffeine can trigger tachycardia and palpitations.

Large or Heavy Meals: Consuming large meals, especially those high in carbohydrates, can increase blood flow to the digestive system and decrease the overall blood volume available for circulation. This postprandial hypotension can significantly exacerbate symptoms of POTS.

Dehydration: Adequate hydration is crucial. Even mild dehydration can decrease blood volume, leading to increased heart rate and blood pooling. Ensuring a regular intake of fluids, particularly water and electrolyte solutions, is essential for symptom management.

Poor Nutrition: Nutritional deficiencies can affect overall health and exacerbate POTS symptoms. Balanced meals with sufficient salt intake (as advised by a healthcare provider) can help in maintaining blood volume and pressure.

Hormonal Fluctuations

Menstrual Cycle and Pregnancy: Many women report a worsening of symptoms during certain phases of their menstrual cycle or pregnancy. Hormonal changes during these times can affect blood volume and vascular tone, leading to more pronounced symptoms.

Puberty and Growth Phases: Adolescents going through growth spurts or puberty may experience an onset or worsening of POTS symptoms due to rapid changes in body size, blood volume, and hormonal levels.

Physical and Emotional Stress

Overexertion: While a graded and well-planned exercise regimen can be beneficial for POTS patients, overdoing physical activities or sudden intense exercise can deplete energy reserves and exacerbate symptoms.

Stress and Anxiety: Psychological stress activates the sympathetic nervous system, potentially worsening tachycardia and other symptoms. Managing stress through techniques such as mindfulness, meditation, or counseling can be an important aspect of managing POTS.

Lack of Regular Exercise: Conversely, a sedentary lifestyle can lead to deconditioning, and worsening orthostatic intolerance. Regular, moderate, and physician-approved exercise is important for maintaining cardiovascular fitness and managing symptoms.

Sleep and Rest Patterns

Poor Sleep Quality and Insomnia: Restful sleep is crucial for overall health particularly so for individuals with POTS. Poor sleep can exacerbate daytime fatigue, cognitive dysfunction, and overall symptom severity.

Prolonged Bed Rest or Inactivity: Extended periods of inactivity, such as bed rest following surgery or illness, can worsen orthostatic intolerance as the body becomes deconditioned to the upright posture. Gradual reconditioning is necessary to avoid a significant exacerbation of symptoms.

Medications

Certain Medications: Various medications can exacerbate POTS symptoms, including some blood pressure medications, diuretics, and even certain supplements. Patients need to discuss all medications and supplements with their healthcare provider to understand potential impacts on their POTS.

Illnesses and Infections

Viral and Bacterial Infections: Infections can act as a trigger for the onset of POTS or exacerbate existing symptoms. The stress of illness on the body, dehydration due to fever or vomiting, and immune system activation can all negatively impact POTS symptomatology.

For individuals with POTS, identifying personal triggers is a process of careful observation and sometimes trial and error. Keeping a detailed symptom diary, noting activities, food and fluid intake, weather, and other potential factors can help in pinpointing what exacerbates symptoms. Collaborating closely with healthcare professionals, including doctors, dietitians, and physical therapists, can aid in developing a comprehensive management plan. This plan may include strategies for avoiding or mitigating triggers, such as lifestyle adjustments, dietary changes, and possibly medication adjustments. Understanding and managing these triggers is a key component in the overall treatment and quality of life improvement for individuals with POTS.

Differentiating POTS from Other Conditions

Differentiating Postural Orthostatic Tachycardia Syndrome (POTS) from other medical conditions with overlapping symptoms is a complex but crucial aspect of diagnosis and treatment. POTS shares commonalities with several disorders, but certain distinguishing features set it apart. Understanding these nuances is vital for clinicians and patients to accurately identify POTS and manage it effectively.

Anxiety and panic disorders often mimic POTS due to similar symptoms like palpitations, rapid heartbeat, and shortness of breath. However, the primary distinction lies in the triggers and patterns of these symptoms. In POTS, symptoms are primarily provoked by an upright posture and are alleviated by lying down. This postural dependency is absent in anxiety disorders, where symptoms typically arise in response to stress or panic triggers and are not directly related to changes in body position.

Orthostatic hypotension (OH) and POTS both involve symptoms that worsen with standing, such as dizziness and lightheadedness. The critical difference is that OH is characterized by a significant drop in blood pressure upon standing. In POTS, the issue is not a substantial decrease in blood pressure, but rather an excessive increase in heart rate without a corresponding drop in blood pressure. Diagnosing OH versus POTS requires careful monitoring of both blood pressure and heart rate in response to postural changes.

Chronic Fatigue Syndrome (CFS) shares the debilitating fatigue and exercise intolerance seen in POTS. However, CFS does not typically include the significant heart rate increase upon standing that is characteristic of POTS. Additionally, while fatigue in CFS is persistent and pervasive, in POTS, it is often more directly linked to physical exertion or prolonged periods in an upright posture.

Vasovagal syncope (VVS) can appear similar to POTS due to fainting or near-fainting episodes common in both conditions. Unlike POTS, VVS usually involves isolated fainting episodes, often triggered by specific stimuli such as emotional distress, prolonged standing, or seeing blood. POTS, on the other hand, is characterized by a consistent pattern of symptoms triggered by standing, with chronic issues rather than episodic fainting.

Dehydration can produce symptoms like dizziness, increased heart rate, and fatigue, similar to those seen in POTS. However, dehydration-related symptoms generally resolve with appropriate fluid intake, whereas POTS symptoms are chronic and tied to postural changes, persisting despite adequate hydration.

Differentiating POTS from other autonomic disorders can be challenging due to the broad range of overlapping symptoms. The hallmark of POTS, however, is its specific pattern of excessive heart rate increase upon standing, which is not common in other autonomic disorders. Accurate diagnosis often involves autonomic function tests, such as the tilt table test, to observe the body's cardiovascular responses to changes in posture.

POTS frequently coexists with other conditions, such as Ehlers-Danlos Syndrome, Mast Cell Activation Syndrome, and various autoimmune disorders. These comorbidities can complicate the presentation and management of POTS. Identifying and addressing these concurrent conditions is essential, as they can significantly impact the overall health and treatment response of POTS patients.

Understanding the unique aspects of POTS and how it differs from other conditions with similar presentations is crucial for accurate diagnosis and effective management. For healthcare providers, this requires a comprehensive evaluation of the patient's symptoms, medical history, and response to postural changes. For patients, knowledge of these distinctions is important for understanding their condition, seeking appropriate care, and advocating for their health in complex medical landscapes.

CHAPTER TWO: MEDICAL MANAGEMENT OF POTS

This chapter provides an overview of the various medications commonly prescribed for POTS, detailing how they function to alleviate symptoms and improve quality of life. We also explore non-pharmacological therapies, such as the use of compression garments and dietary modifications like increased salt intake, which play a pivotal role in managing this condition. Understanding the importance of a collaborative approach to healthcare, we offer guidance on effectively communicating with medical professionals and building a supportive healthcare team.

Additionally, we navigate the intricacies of the healthcare system, providing practical advice on handling insurance issues, locating specialized care, and advocating for comprehensive and personalized treatment. This chapter is designed to empower patients and caregivers with knowledge and strategies for navigating the complex journey of managing POTS.

Medications and Their Role

Managing Postural Orthostatic Tachycardia Syndrome (POTS) often involves the use of various medications. These drugs play a significant role in alleviating symptoms, improving quality of life, and addressing the underlying physiological dysfunctions associated with POTS. Here is a detailed overview of the common medications used in POTS treatment and their mechanisms of action:

Beta-Blockers

Beta-blockers such as Propranolol, Metoprolol, and Atenolol are standard in POTS treatment. They work by blocking the beta-adrenergic receptors in the heart and blood vessels, which reduces the effects of adrenaline. This decrease in adrenaline activity results in a slower heart rate and reduced force of heart contractions, effectively controlling the tachycardia that characterizes POTS. While these medications are beneficial in managing palpitations, chest discomfort, and rapid heartbeats, they must be prescribed cautiously due to potential side effects like fatigue, dizziness, and respiratory issues. The choice and dosage of a specific beta-blocker are tailored to each patient based on their symptom profile and overall health.

Fludrocortisone

Fludrocortisone is a synthetic corticosteroid that acts on the kidneys to increase sodium retention, leading to an increase in blood volume. For POTS patients, this is particularly advantageous as it counteracts the blood pooling and orthostatic hypotension often observed in the condition. By boosting blood volume, Fludrocortisone reduces symptoms such as dizziness and syncope associated with standing. However, it is important to monitor for side effects like fluid retention, hypertension, and low potassium levels. Dietary adjustments and monitoring are crucial for patients taking Fludrocortisone to manage these risks effectively.

Midodrine

Midodrine is an alpha-1 adrenoreceptor agonist, meaning it increases vascular tone by constricting blood vessels, thus increasing blood pressure. It is specifically beneficial in reducing orthostatic blood pooling and improving cerebral blood flow in POTS patients, which helps in alleviating symptoms of lightheadedness and syncope upon standing. However, Midodrine must be used judiciously to prevent supine hypertension, and patients are advised to avoid lying down immediately after taking it. The timing of Midodrine administration is critical to ensure that it provides maximum benefit during the daytime when the patient is most active.

Ivabradine

Ivabradine specifically targets the sinoatrial node of the heart to reduce heart rate, making it an excellent option for POTS patients with high heart rates that are not adequately controlled by beta-blockers. By selectively inhibiting the I_f channels, Ivabradine slows down the heart rate without significantly affecting blood pressure. This can be particularly beneficial for patients whose primary symptom is tachycardia. However, patients on Ivabradine need to be monitored for side effects such as visual disturbances and too low a heart rate.

SSRIs and SNRIs

Selective Serotonin Reuptake Inhibitors (SSRIs) and Serotonin-Norepinephrine Reuptake Inhibitors (SNRIs) like Sertraline and Venlafaxine are sometimes used in POTS treatment. These antidepressants are thought to regulate the autonomic nervous system. They are particularly beneficial in managing underlying anxiety or depression often associated with chronic conditions like POTS. While they may help stabilize heart rate and blood pressure, starting doses should be low and gradually increased. Monitoring for side effects, including gastrointestinal disturbances, sexual dysfunction, and sleep issues, is essential for patients on these medications.

Pyridostigmine

Pyridostigmine, a cholinesterase inhibitor, enhances the action of acetylcholine, a neurotransmitter that promotes muscle contraction and communication between nerves and muscles. By improving muscle tone in blood vessels, it potentially enhances vascular response and can reduce orthostatic tachycardia in POTS patients. Pyridostigmine is usually well-tolerated and can be particularly beneficial for those who haven't found relief with other treatments. However, its use should be monitored for potential gastrointestinal side effects like cramping and diarrhea.

In addition to these primary medications, treatment for POTS may include other drugs for symptom-specific management, such as antihistamines for patients with mast cell activation symptoms or gastrointestinal prokinetics for those with digestive issues.

The appropriate medication regimen for a POTS patient is highly individualized. The choice and combination of medications depend on the patient's symptom profile, response to initial treatments, and coexisting conditions. Regular follow-ups and possible adjustments to the medication plan are essential, as POTS symptoms can change over time. Patients should be educated about potential side effects and the importance of medication adherence. The overarching goal of pharmacotherapy in POTS is not only to reduce symptoms but also to enhance the patient's ability to engage in daily activities and improve overall life quality.

Non-Pharmacological Therapies

In managing Postural Orthostatic Tachycardia Syndrome (POTS), non-pharmacological therapies are as crucial as medications. These therapies focus on lifestyle changes, physical strategies, and dietary adjustments to alleviate symptoms and improve the overall quality of life for individuals with POTS. Here's a detailed overview of various non-pharmacological treatments for POTS:

Increased Salt and Fluid Intake

One of the fundamental non-pharmacological recommendations for POTS patients is to increase salt and fluid intake. This strategy aims to boost blood volume, counteracting the low blood volume (hypovolemia) often seen in POTS. Patients are typically advised to consume a higher-than-average amount of salt and to increase their fluid intake, focusing on water and electrolyte-rich beverages. This approach can be particularly effective in reducing symptoms like dizziness, fatigue, and syncope. However, it's essential to monitor blood pressure, as excessive salt intake may not be suitable for all patients, especially those with hypertension.

Compression Garments

Compression garments, including stockings and abdominal binders, are another key non-pharmacological treatment for POTS. These garments exert pressure on the lower body and abdomen, reducing the orthostatic pooling of blood in these areas. By preventing blood from accumulating excessively in the legs and abdomen, compression garments can significantly alleviate symptoms such as lightheadedness and fainting. Patients should choose the right type of compression garment (knee-high, thigh-high, or full-length) and the appropriate level of compression, ensuring a proper fit for maximum efficacy.

Physical Therapy and Exercise

Regular exercise is highly beneficial in managing POTS, as it can enhance cardiovascular fitness and strengthen the autonomic nervous system. However, the type of exercise is crucial. Recumbent exercises, such as rowing, swimming, or cycling, are often recommended because they are less likely to trigger orthostatic symptoms compared to upright exercises. Gradual and consistent exercise routines, developed with the guidance of a physical therapist, can help patients build tolerance and improve symptoms over time. Physical therapists can also provide tailored exercise programs and offer advice on managing symptoms during physical activities.

Dietary Adjustments

Dietary adjustments can play a significant role in managing POTS. Eating smaller, more frequent meals can help prevent the significant blood pooling that often occurs after larger meals (postprandial hypotension). Additionally, some patients might benefit from specific dietary modifications, such as a gluten-free diet if they have gluten sensitivity, which can exacerbate POTS symptoms. Maintaining a balanced diet, rich in nutrients, is also important for overall health and well-being.

Adequate Sleep and Sleep Hygiene

Good quality sleep is crucial for POTS patients. Poor sleep can exacerbate symptoms like fatigue and cognitive dysfunction. Implementing good sleep hygiene practices, such as maintaining a consistent sleep schedule, creating a comfortable and conducive sleep environment, and avoiding stimulants like caffeine before bedtime, can enhance sleep quality. Additionally, some patients may find relief from POTS symptoms in the morning by slightly elevating the head of their bed, which can promote better blood volume regulation during sleep.

Stress Management

Managing emotional stress is vital in POTS treatment, as stress can trigger or worsen symptoms by stimulating the sympathetic nervous system. Techniques like yoga, meditation, deep breathing exercises, and mindfulness can be effective tools for managing stress. These practices not only help in reducing stress-related symptoms but also contribute to overall emotional well-being.

Avoiding Triggers

Identifying and avoiding triggers that exacerbate POTS symptoms is a key aspect of management. Common triggers include standing for long periods, exposure to hot environments, and consuming certain foods and beverages, like alcohol or caffeine. Implementing lifestyle modifications, such as taking breaks to sit down, using cooling devices in hot weather, and moderating dietary triggers, can help manage symptoms effectively.

Patient Education and Support

Educating patients about POTS, its symptoms, and management strategies is critical. Understanding the condition empowers patients to take an active role in their care. Additionally, participating in support groups can provide emotional support and practical tips from others who are experiencing similar challenges. Peer support can be a valuable resource in coping with the daily challenges of living with POTS.

Non-pharmacological therapies for POTS require a commitment to lifestyle changes and proactive self-care. These strategies are often personalized based on each patient's symptoms and lifestyle, and their effectiveness can be enhanced when used in conjunction with pharmacological treatments. Regular consultations with healthcare providers are important to ensure that these non-pharmacological approaches are effective and to make adjustments as needed.

Working with Healthcare Professionals

Effectively managing Postural Orthostatic Tachycardia Syndrome (POTS) requires a proactive approach to working with healthcare professionals. Establishing a strong, communicative relationship with your medical team is essential for receiving the best possible care. Below is a detailed guide on how to effectively communicate with doctors and build a supportive healthcare team for POTS management.

Establishing a Good Patient-Doctor Relationship

Creating a strong rapport with your healthcare providers is foundational. Open and honest communication about your symptoms, lifestyle, and concerns is crucial. Before each appointment, prepare a list of symptoms, changes in your condition, and any questions or concerns you have. This preparation can help make your appointments more productive. Keeping a detailed symptom diary can also be incredibly helpful, providing your doctor with a clear picture of your day-to-day experiences. Additionally, educating yourself about POTS and its management can empower you to have more informed discussions with your healthcare team.

Building a Multi-disciplinary Team

POTS can affect various systems in the body, so it's often beneficial to have a multi-disciplinary team. This team may include a cardiologist, neurologist, primary care physician, and specialists like physical therapists, dietitians, or psychologists. Ensuring that these professionals are willing to communicate and collaborate is vital for a coordinated approach to your care. Each specialist brings a unique perspective and expertise, contributing to a comprehensive treatment plan.

Effective Communication Strategies

Effective communication with your healthcare providers is key. Be clear and concise when describing your symptoms and the impact they have on your daily life. Don't hesitate to ask questions about your diagnosis, treatment options, and prognosis. This not only helps you understand your condition better but also ensures that you are fully informed about your care. Additionally, provide feedback on your treatments, including any side effects or challenges you're facing. This feedback is essential for your doctors to tailor your treatment plan effectively.

Advocating for Yourself

Self-advocacy is important, especially if you feel your concerns are not being fully addressed. If necessary, seek second opinions or ask for referrals to specialists. Be aware of your rights as a patient, including access to your medical records and the right to privacy. Understanding your health insurance coverage is also crucial, as it determines what treatments and medications are accessible to you.

Addressing Mental Health

Managing a chronic condition like POTS can take a toll on your mental health. Be open with your healthcare providers about any mental health challenges you're facing. They can provide referrals to mental health services, such as counseling or therapy, which can be an integral part of your overall treatment plan. Additionally, consider joining support groups for individuals with POTS. These groups provide emotional encouragement, useful guidance, and a feeling of belonging.

In summary, working effectively with healthcare professionals when managing POTS involves clear communication, thorough preparation, and active participation in your care. Building a multi-disciplinary team and advocating for your needs are key components of successful management. Additionally, addressing the mental and emotional aspects of living with POTS is crucial for comprehensive care. Remember, you are an important member of your healthcare team, and your engagement and input are vital to your treatment and well-being.

Navigating the Healthcare System

Navigating the healthcare system while managing a condition like Postural Orthostatic Tachycardia Syndrome (POTS) can be complex and overwhelming. It involves understanding insurance policies, finding the right specialists, and advocating effectively for your care. Here's an in-depth guide on how to navigate these aspects:

Understanding and Managing Insurance

Know Your Policy: Begin by thoroughly understanding your health insurance policy. Familiarize yourself with what treatments, medications, and specialist visits are covered. Pay special attention to details like co-pays, deductibles, out-of-pocket maximums, and coverage limitations.

Regular Review: Insurance policies and coverage can change. It's important to regularly review your policy and stay informed about any changes that could impact your care.

Handling Pre-Authorizations: Certain treatments or specialist visits might require pre-authorization from your insurance provider. Understand this process, as failure to get pre-authorization can result in denied claims. Keep track of all communications and authorizations for your records.

Appealing Denials: If your insurance denies a claim or coverage for a specific treatment, familiarize yourself with the appeal process. Document all interactions and collect necessary information such as medical records, letters from healthcare providers, and a clear explanation of why the treatment is necessary. Persistence is key in appealing insurance decisions.

Finding the Right Specialists

Research Specialists: Finding specialists who are knowledgeable about POTS is critical. Research doctors and medical centers that specialize in autonomic disorders or have a track record of treating POTS patients.

Utilize Referrals: Referrals from your primary care physician can be a valuable pathway to finding the right specialist. A referral can also sometimes expedite the process of getting an appointment.

Online Resources: Online forums, patient advocacy groups, and POTS community websites can be excellent resources for recommendations on specialists.

Prepare for Visits: When visiting a specialist, come prepared with your medical history, a list of current medications, and a summary of your symptoms. Being well-prepared can maximize the effectiveness of your consultation.

Advocating for Care

Self-Advocacy: Advocating for yourself is crucial. This means being assertive in asking questions, seeking second opinions when necessary, and discussing all possible treatment options.

Effective Communication: Develop effective communication skills to convey your needs, symptoms, and treatment preferences to your healthcare providers. Be clear about the challenges you're facing, including any barriers in accessing care or medications.

Support Networks: Building a support network, including family, and friends, or connecting with patient advocacy groups, can provide additional support and resources in navigating the healthcare system.

Know Your Rights: Educate yourself about your legal rights as a patient. This includes the right to access your medical records, privacy rights under HIPAA, and your right to informed consent regarding treatments.

Coordinating Care

Organization: With POTS often requiring consultations with multiple specialists, organization is key. Keep a detailed health diary or a binder with records of all your medical appointments, treatments, test results, and doctor's recommendations.

Communication Between Providers: Encourage open communication between your various healthcare providers. This might involve signing releases to allow different doctors to share your medical information, ensuring everyone involved in your care is on the same page.

Navigating the healthcare system effectively requires being informed, organized, and proactive. Understanding your insurance plan, identifying the right specialists, advocating for your needs, and coordinating your care are all vital components of effectively managing POTS. Empowering yourself with knowledge and maintaining open lines of communication with your healthcare providers and insurance companies are critical steps in receiving the best possible care.

CHAPTER THREE: LIFESTYLE ADJUSTMENTS FOR POTS

This chapter focuses on essential lifestyle changes and strategies beneficial for individuals with Postural Orthostatic Tachycardia Syndrome (POTS). It covers the significance of diet and nutrition, providing guidelines for dietary adjustments that can alleviate POTS symptoms. The chapter also discusses safe exercise routines and approaches to gradually increase physical activity, tailored to the needs of those with POTS.

Emphasizing the importance of rest and sleep hygiene, it explores how proper sleep management is crucial in controlling symptoms. Additionally, it offers practical advice for managing orthostatic intolerance, including techniques for coping with standing and adapting to positional changes, all aimed at improving the overall quality of life for POTS patients.

Diet and Nutrition

Managing Postural Orthostatic Tachycardia Syndrome (POTS) effectively often involves making significant dietary and nutritional adjustments. These changes can help alleviate some of the symptoms associated with POTS by stabilizing blood volume and blood pressure, managing energy levels, and improving overall bodily functions. Here is an extended, detailed guide on dietary modifications beneficial for POTS patients:

Increased Salt Intake

For many individuals with POTS, increasing salt intake is a key dietary change. Salt aids in water retention within the body, which in turn boosts the volume of blood. This can be particularly helpful in reducing symptoms like lightheadedness and fainting, which are often due to low blood volume in POTS. Incorporating more salt can be achieved through adding salt to foods, consuming salty snacks, or using salt tablets, as recommended by a healthcare provider. It's essential to consult a doctor before increasing salt intake, especially for those with conditions like hypertension or heart disease, where high salt intake might be contraindicated.

Adequate Hydration

Hydration is critically important for POTS patients. Maintaining adequate fluid levels helps in sustaining blood volume and preventing blood pressure drops. Patients are generally advised to drink at least 2-3 liters of fluids daily. This can include water, electrolyte-replenishing beverages, and herbal teas. Caffeine and alcohol, which can be dehydrating, should be consumed in moderation or avoided, as they can exacerbate POTS symptoms.

Small, Frequent Meals

Large meals can trigger POTS symptoms by redirecting blood flow to the digestive system, away from the heart and brain. To counter this, eating smaller, more frequent meals throughout the day is recommended. This approach helps in managing blood flow and maintaining stable energy levels. It also reduces the risk of postprandial hypotension, a drop in blood pressure following meals, which is common in POTS patients.

Balanced Diet

A balanced diet is essential for managing POTS. This involves incorporating a diverse selection of fruits, vegetables, whole grains, lean protein sources, and beneficial fats into one's diet. Such a diet provides necessary nutrients and helps in overall health maintenance. Some POTS patients may experience food intolerances or sensitivities, such as gluten or dairy. Keeping a food diary to track how certain foods affect symptoms can be insightful. It can guide dietary choices and identify any specific foods to avoid.

Limiting Refined Carbohydrates and Sugars

Foods high in refined carbohydrates and sugars can cause rapid fluctuations in blood sugar levels. These fluctuations can exacerbate POTS symptoms by causing energy spikes and crashes. Opting for foods with complex carbohydrates and a low glycemic index, such as whole grains, legumes, and some fruits, can help maintain steady blood sugar levels, providing more consistent energy throughout the day.

Increasing Fiber Intake

A high-fiber diet can benefit POTS patients, particularly those experiencing gastrointestinal issues, which are common with the condition. Fiber aids in digestive health and can help regulate bowel movements. Vegetables, fruits, whole grains, and legumes are examples of foods that are high in fiber. However, it's important to increase fiber intake gradually to prevent gastrointestinal discomfort.

Managing Orthostatic Intolerance Through Diet

Alongside increased salt and fluid intake, identifying and avoiding foods and drinks that trigger or worsen orthostatic intolerance is important. This may include stimulants like caffeine or specific foods that individual patients find aggravating. Each person with POTS may have different triggers, so personal observation and adjustment are key.

Nutritional Supplements

Certain nutritional supplements may be beneficial for POTS patients, especially if they have specific deficiencies. Supplements such as magnesium, which can aid in muscle function and blood pressure regulation, vitamin B12, and iron might be recommended, but only under the guidance of a healthcare professional.

Professional Nutritional Guidance

Given the complexities of POTS and the individual variations in symptoms and triggers, consulting with a dietitian or nutritionist who has experience with POTS can be extremely beneficial. They can provide personalized advice, and tailored meal plans, and help navigate any specific dietary needs or restrictions.

In summary, dietary and nutritional adjustments are integral components of managing POTS. An individualized approach, focusing on hydration, balanced and smaller meals, and careful monitoring of food triggers and nutrient intake, is essential. Regular consultations with healthcare and nutritional professionals are advisable to ensure that these dietary strategies are effective and in line with overall health goals.

Exercise and Physical Activity

Exercise and physical activity are essential in managing Postural Orthostatic Tachycardia Syndrome (POTS), but it's important to approach them with caution and awareness of how the body responds. For POTS patients, initiating an exercise routine starts with low-impact activities. These activities, like recumbent biking, rowing, or swimming, are chosen for their minimal impact on the cardiovascular system, particularly in terms of mitigating the gravitational stress that can exacerbate POTS symptoms. The goal in these initial stages is to engage in exercises that keep the body in a horizontal or semi-horizontal position, reducing the likelihood of triggering symptoms such as rapid heart rate, dizziness, or fainting spells.

When beginning an exercise regimen, POTS patients are advised to start with short, manageable sessions – sometimes as brief as 5-10 minutes per day – and at a very low intensity. The key is to ensure that these activities do not provoke POTS symptoms significantly. As the body begins to adapt to these exercise routines, the duration and intensity can be gradually increased. This could mean extending exercise sessions by a few minutes each week or gently increasing the resistance or speed at which exercises are performed. The progression should be slow and entirely based on the individual's tolerance, as rushing this process can lead to setbacks in symptom management.

As physical tolerance improves, incorporating strength training exercises can offer additional benefits. Building muscle strength, especially in the legs and core, can help improve blood circulation and overall stamina, factors that are crucial in managing POTS. Initial strength training should focus on exercises that can be performed while seated or lying down, using light weights or resistance bands. These exercises help in targeting major muscle groups without placing undue strain on the body.

The progression to more upright exercises is a significant milestone in a POTS patient's exercise journey. This transition must be gradual and closely monitored. Simple activities like walking or light jogging can be introduced slowly. Yoga and Pilates are also beneficial as they combine strength, flexibility, and balance training. However, individuals with POTS need to be prepared to adapt these exercises, or even stop them temporarily if they notice an exacerbation of symptoms.

Maintaining a consistent exercise routine is vital, but so is recognizing the need for rest and recovery. Regular exercise is ideal, but it must be balanced with the body's need for rest to avoid overexertion. Overdoing exercise can exacerbate POTS symptoms, so it's crucial to listen to the body and incorporate rest days as needed. Documenting exercise routines, along with any changes in symptoms, is a practical approach to track progress and identify patterns. This record-keeping can provide valuable insights into how different exercises impact symptoms, helping to fine-tune the exercise regimen.

For personalized guidance, working with physical therapists or exercise physiologists who have experience with POTS can be highly beneficial. These professionals can assist in developing tailored exercise programs, provide advice on how to safely increase physical activity, and offer strategies to manage symptoms during exercise. They can also help monitor progress and make necessary adjustments to exercise routines, ensuring they align with the individual's changing needs and capabilities.

In conclusion, a carefully planned, gradually intensified exercise program is essential for managing POTS effectively. Starting with low-impact, recumbent exercises and slowly introducing strength training and more upright activities can lead to significant improvements in managing POTS symptoms. Consistent monitoring, adaptation based on individual response, and professional guidance are key to successfully incorporating exercise into the lifestyle of someone living with POTS.

Sleep and Rest

Managing sleep and rest is a vital aspect of living with Postural Orthostatic Tachycardia Syndrome (POTS), as these elements significantly impact the severity and management of the condition. For individuals with POTS, understanding and implementing effective sleep hygiene and rest strategies can play a critical role in alleviating symptoms and enhancing overall quality of life. Here's a detailed exploration of the importance of rest and sleep hygiene for POTS patients:

The Crucial Role of Rest in POTS Management

Rest is an essential component in managing POTS. The nature of this condition often results in chronic fatigue, which can be debilitating. Integrating regular rest periods into daily routines can significantly help in managing this fatigue. These rest periods, especially when taken in a reclined or horizontal position, can alleviate the orthostatic stress that exacerbates POTS symptoms. Rest allows the body to recover and repair, reducing the workload on the heart and circulatory system. For POTS patients, even short periods of rest throughout the day can make a substantial difference in symptom management and overall energy levels.

The Importance of Sleep Hygiene

Good sleep hygiene is critical for POTS patients, as poor sleep can exacerbate symptoms and disrupt the autonomic nervous system's function. Establishing a regular sleep routine is vital in regulating the body's internal clock. Consistent sleep and wake times, including on weekends, help stabilize the circadian rhythm, leading to improved sleep quality. The sleep environment should be optimized for restfulness, with a comfortable mattress and pillows, a cool room temperature, and minimal noise and light. Blackout curtains, eye masks, and earplugs may be necessary for some individuals to create an environment conducive to sleep.

Sleep Positioning Strategies for POTS

Many POTS patients find relief from symptoms by adjusting their sleeping positions. Elevating the head of the bed slightly can reduce symptoms like morning lightheadedness and rapid heartbeat, as this position aids in better blood volume regulation during sleep. Using pillows to find a comfortable and supportive sleep position can also be beneficial. For instance, placing pillows under the legs can improve circulation and reduce discomfort.

Tackling Sleep Disturbances

Sleep disturbances, including insomnia and disrupted sleep patterns, are common among POTS patients. Practicing relaxation techniques before bedtime, such as deep breathing exercises, meditation, or gentle yoga, can help prepare the body and mind for sleep. Limiting the intake of stimulants like caffeine, particularly in the latter part of the day, is essential for improving sleep quality. Additionally, avoiding heavy meals, intense exercise, or stimulating activities close to bedtime can prevent sleep disruptions.

The Strategic Use of Napping

While daytime naps can be beneficial in managing fatigue for POTS patients, they should be used strategically. Long or late afternoon naps can interfere with nighttime sleep patterns. Short, restorative naps earlier in the day are generally more beneficial and less likely to disrupt night-time sleep.

Seeking Professional Help for Sleep Issues

Persistent sleep issues should be addressed with the help of healthcare professionals. Conditions such as sleep apnea, restless leg syndrome, or other sleep-related disorders are not uncommon in individuals with POTS and can significantly impact sleep quality. A healthcare provider can offer guidance on appropriate treatments, sleep studies, or interventions necessary to improve sleep.

In summary, effective management of sleep and rest is key for individuals with POTS. Implementing good sleep hygiene, optimizing the sleep environment, addressing sleep disturbances, and incorporating regular rest periods can profoundly impact the management of POTS symptoms. Regular evaluation and adaptation of these practices, in consultation with healthcare providers, are crucial to ensure they are effectively aiding in the management of the condition.

Managing Orthostatic Intolerance

Effectively managing orthostatic intolerance, a key challenge for individuals with Postural Orthostatic Tachycardia Syndrome (POTS), requires a comprehensive approach that addresses the difficulties experienced with standing and positional changes.

Orthostatic intolerance can manifest as a range of symptoms, including dizziness, rapid heart rate, fainting, and lightheadedness, making everyday activities challenging. To alleviate these symptoms, several strategies can be employed.

One of the fundamental approaches is to make slow and deliberate transitions between positions. For instance, when moving from a lying to a standing position, it's advisable to first sit up and pause for a few moments, allowing the body to adapt to the change in posture. This gradual process can help the circulatory system adjust to the new position, reducing the risk of symptoms like dizziness or lightheadedness. Similarly, rising slowly from a sitting position to standing can help prevent sudden drops in blood pressure.

Physical counter-maneuvers are effective techniques for POTS patients to manage orthostatic intolerance. These maneuvers involve actions like crossing the legs and tensing thigh muscles, squatting, or clenching fists, which can increase blood pressure temporarily and improve blood flow to the heart and brain. These actions are particularly useful during prolonged standing or when symptoms of lightheadedness begin to emerge.

The use of compression garments, such as compression stockings or abdominal binders, is another key strategy. These garments provide support to the blood vessels, helping to push blood upwards and reduce pooling in the lower extremities. The effectiveness of compression garments depends on the correct level of pressure and fit, so it's important to consult with a healthcare professional to find the most suitable type for individual needs.

Maintaining adequate hydration and an appropriate level of salt intake is also crucial in managing orthostatic intolerance. Staying well-hydrated helps maintain blood volume, which is essential for preventing drops in blood pressure upon standing. Increased salt intake can have a similar effect by retaining more fluid in the body, but this should be balanced with overall health considerations, especially for those with conditions like hypertension. A healthcare provider can offer guidance on the right balance of fluid and salt intake for individual cases.

Leg elevation can provide immediate relief for some POTS patients experiencing symptoms of orthostatic intolerance. This can involve elevating the legs while sitting or lying down to facilitate venous return to the heart. This simple technique can be especially beneficial when symptoms such as lightheadedness or pre-syncope are felt.

Pacing and planning daily activities is crucial. Understanding personal limits and avoiding overexertion can prevent exacerbation of symptoms. Scheduling demanding activities at times when symptoms are typically less severe and incorporating regular rest breaks can help manage energy levels more effectively.

Regular exercise, especially routines focusing on leg and core strength, can improve blood circulation over time and reduce symptoms of orthostatic intolerance. However, exercise programs should be tailored to individual capabilities and symptoms, and it's often beneficial to work with a physical therapist or exercise specialist familiar with POTS. They can develop a safe and effective exercise plan, gradually increasing intensity and duration as tolerance improves.

In some instances, medications may be prescribed as part of the management strategy for orthostatic intolerance. These can include drugs to increase blood volume, regulate blood pressure, or improve heart function. Regular medical consultations are important to monitor the condition, adjust medications as needed, and ensure comprehensive care.

In summary, managing orthostatic intolerance in POTS requires a multifaceted approach that includes careful positional changes, physical counter-maneuvers, the use of compression garments, maintaining hydration and appropriate salt intake, leg elevation, pacing daily activities, regular exercise, and potential medication. Each strategy plays a role in alleviating the challenges posed by orthostatic intolerance, enhancing the ability to perform daily activities with greater comfort and stability. Regular follow-up with healthcare professionals is essential to ensure that these management strategies are effectively tailored to individual needs and health considerations.

CHAPTER FOUR: COPING STRATEGIES AND SUPPORT SYSTEMS

This chapter explores the essential approaches for managing Postural Orthostatic Tachycardia Syndrome (POTS). It delves into the psychological impact of POTS, discussing mental health challenges and providing practical stress management and coping strategies. The chapter emphasizes the importance of building a supportive network, highlighting how support groups, online communities, and family support can play pivotal roles in managing the condition.

It also offers resources for education and advocacy, empowering patients to raise awareness about POTS. Additionally, the chapter outlines strategies for long-term management, including adapting to lifestyle changes and planning for continuous care, essential for enhancing the quality of life with POTS.

Psychological Impact and Coping Mechanisms

Living with Postural Orthostatic Tachycardia Syndrome (POTS) involves navigating not only physical symptoms but also significant psychological challenges. The chronic nature of POTS, characterized by symptoms like dizziness, fatigue, and heart palpitations, can have a profound impact on mental health, necessitating robust coping strategies and mental health support.

Psychological Impact of POTS

Individuals with POTS often grapple with mental health challenges such as anxiety, depression, and chronic stress. These issues stem partly from the unpredictable and debilitating nature of POTS symptoms, which can disrupt daily life, social activities, and work. The uncertainty and chronicity of the condition can foster feelings of frustration, helplessness, and a loss of control over one's life, contributing to emotional distress. Additionally, the physical limitations imposed by POTS can lead to social isolation, exacerbating feelings of loneliness and disconnection, and further impacting mental health.

Stress Management in POTS

Stress management is a critical component of living with POTS, as stress can trigger or worsen physical symptoms. Identifying personal stressors is crucial, as it allows individuals to develop specific strategies to manage them effectively. Techniques such as deep breathing exercises, meditation, mindfulness practices, and gentle yoga can be highly beneficial. These practices not only aid in reducing stress but also have positive physiological effects, promoting relaxation and improving autonomic function. Establishing a structured daily routine, including consistent sleep patterns and dedicated relaxation or mindfulness sessions, can instill a sense of predictability and control, which is often lacking for those with POTS.

Coping Strategies for Mental Health

Cognitive-Behavioral Therapy (CBT): Cognitive-Behavioral Therapy is particularly effective for POTS patients. It focuses on altering negative thoughts and behaviors associated with chronic illness, fostering resilience and adaptive coping mechanisms. Through CBT, patients can learn to manage the psychological aspects of POTS more effectively, enhancing overall well-being.

Counseling and Psychotherapy: Regular counseling or psychotherapy sessions offer a supportive environment to discuss the emotional and psychological challenges of living with POTS. Therapists can assist in addressing issues such as anxiety, depression, and the stress associated with chronic illness.

Support Groups and Community Engagement: Participating in support groups specifically for POTS, either online or in person, provides an opportunity to connect with others who face similar challenges. Sharing experiences and coping strategies in a supportive community can reduce feelings of isolation and provide practical tips for managing the condition.

Lifestyle Considerations for Mental Health

Incorporating lifestyle changes can significantly aid in managing the mental health aspects of POTS. Regular, POTS-friendly physical activities, such as light walking, swimming, or recumbent cycling, can improve mood and alleviate stress by releasing endorphins. Balancing a healthy diet and ensuring consistent, quality sleep are also important for mental well-being. These lifestyle adjustments can have a positive impact on both physical and mental health, contributing to better overall management of POTS.

Professional Mental Health Support

Seeking professional mental health support is crucial for individuals with POTS experiencing significant psychological difficulties. Mental health professionals can provide tailored treatment plans, which may include medication for managing anxiety or depressive symptoms. Regular consultations with healthcare professionals ensure that both the physical and psychological aspects of POTS are adequately addressed, forming a comprehensive approach to treatment.

In summary, addressing the psychological impact of POTS is as important as managing its physical symptoms. Implementing stress management techniques, engaging in psychological therapies, participating in supportive communities, making lifestyle adjustments, and seeking professional mental health support are all key elements in managing the condition. A holistic approach that encompasses both physical and psychological care is essential for improving the quality of life for individuals living with POTS.

Building a Support Network

Building a strong support network is crucial for individuals living with Postural Orthostatic Tachycardia Syndrome (POTS), as it provides essential emotional, informational, and practical support. Support groups, in particular, offer a space where individuals can share experiences and coping strategies, fostering a sense of belonging and understanding. Finding the right support group can involve reaching out to local health organizations, hospitals, or national POTS associations. Regular attendance and active participation in these groups can be immensely therapeutic, offering different perspectives on managing POTS and reinforcing a sense of community.

Online communities also play a vital role in expanding the support network for POTS patients. These platforms provide access to a diverse group of individuals and are especially beneficial for those without access to local support groups or who prefer the convenience of online interaction. Social media groups, dedicated health forums, and specialized websites offer spaces for individuals with POTS to connect, share advice, and find support. These online communities are also valuable sources of information, keeping members informed about the latest research, treatments, and management strategies for POTS.

Family support is another critical component of a robust support system for individuals with POTS. Family members can provide unparalleled emotional support, practical assistance with daily activities, and a compassionate understanding of the challenges faced. Educating family members about POTS, its symptoms, and its impact is crucial. This understanding enables them to provide more effective and empathetic support. Open communication about the needs and limitations associated with POTS is key to creating a supportive and accommodating home environment.

In addition to peer and family support, nurturing individual relationships is important. Personal connections with friends, fellow POTS patients, or supportive family members offer tailored advice and a deeper level of emotional understanding. These one-on-one relationships can provide specific insights and strategies that are particularly relevant to an individual's unique experience with POTS.

Professional guidance from therapists or counselors experienced in chronic illness can also be invaluable. They offer coping strategies and psychological support tailored to the challenges of living with a chronic condition like POTS. Engaging with a therapist can provide a structured approach to addressing the emotional and psychological aspects of POTS, complementing the support received from groups, online communities, and family.

In conclusion, a comprehensive support network for POTS patients should ideally encompass support groups, online communities, family support, personal relationships, and professional guidance. Each element of this network offers unique benefits, and together, they provide a multifaceted system of support essential for managing the complexities of living with POTS. Regular and active engagement with this support network can significantly enhance the quality of life and overall well-being of individuals affected by POTS.

Educational and Advocacy Resources

Gaining comprehensive knowledge and actively participating in advocacy is crucial for individuals dealing with Postural Orthostatic Tachycardia Syndrome (POTS). Understanding the condition deeply and helping others learn about it empowers patients, fosters a supportive community, and contributes to the broader goal of increasing recognition and understanding of POTS in the medical community and the general public.

The foundation of managing POTS effectively lies in understanding the condition thoroughly. This includes learning about its symptoms, diagnosis processes, treatment options, and day-to-day management techniques. Reliable sources for educational materials include medical journals, healthcare provider resources, POTS-focused websites, and patient advocacy organizations. These resources can offer a wide spectrum of information from scientific research articles and clinical studies to patient guides and tips for daily living.

For instance, detailed articles explaining the physiological mechanisms of POTS or personal stories from other patients can provide both scientific understanding and practical insights. Additionally, webinars, podcasts, and video content created by healthcare professionals or experienced patients can be beneficial for visual and auditory learners.

Raising awareness about POTS is a continuous need as it helps in increasing public understanding, improving patient care, and potentially influencing healthcare policy. Sharing personal experiences with POTS through social media, blogs, or community events can help in humanizing the condition and spreading awareness. Individuals can also participate in or organize awareness campaigns during specific events like POTS awareness day or related health observances. Engaging with local media to feature stories about living with POTS or the latest research can further broaden the reach of advocacy efforts.

Networking and collaborating with existing advocacy groups and organizations is also vital. These groups often lead larger campaigns, engage in lobbying for policy changes, and provide resources for new advocates to get involved. Advocates can work towards various goals, such as increasing research funding for POTS, improving clinical training for healthcare providers, or advocating for patient rights and accommodations in various settings, including workplaces and educational institutions.

Creating and participating in educational workshops, seminars, and webinars is an effective way to disseminate knowledge about POTS. These can be targeted at different audiences - patients and their families, healthcare professionals, or the general community. Well-informed patients can lead or participate in these sessions, sharing their knowledge and experiences, and answering questions from attendees. This not only helps to educate others but also empowers patients by giving them an active role in the POTS community.

Support groups play a critical role in the educational and emotional support of POTS patients. These groups can be platforms for sharing the latest information about POTS management, treatment innovations, and personal coping strategies. The support group meetings, whether in-person or virtual, provide a space for individuals to express their concerns, learn from others' experiences, and feel less isolated in their journey with POTS.

Facilitating or participating in these groups can significantly enhance the support network available to individuals affected by POTS.

While individual and community efforts are invaluable, professional guidance from therapists, educators, or patient advocates experienced in chronic illness can enhance the effectiveness of educational and advocacy efforts. These professionals can provide structured educational materials, help in designing advocacy campaigns, or offer counseling and support strategies tailored to the needs of POTS patients. They can also assist in navigating the healthcare system, understanding patient rights, and advocating for appropriate medical care and accommodations.

In conclusion, a comprehensive approach to education and advocacy is essential for effectively managing POTS and enhancing awareness about the condition. Deepening personal understanding, actively engaging in community education, participating in advocacy efforts, and leveraging professional guidance are all integral to this approach. By embracing these strategies, individuals with POTS, along with their supporters and healthcare professionals, can contribute to a more informed, empathetic, and supportive environment for all those affected by POTS.

Long-term Management Strategies

Long-term management of Postural Orthostatic Tachycardia Syndrome (POTS) requires an approach that is both comprehensive and adaptable, given the condition's complex and fluctuating nature. It involves a consistent and informed effort to manage not just the physical symptoms, but also the emotional and practical aspects of living with a chronic illness.

Accepting POTS as a chronic condition is foundational to its management. This acceptance helps in setting realistic expectations and understanding that the journey may include periods of fluctuation in symptoms and varying levels of intensity. Individuals with POTS need to recognize that some days will be better than others and that adjustments in management strategies may be necessary over time.

Ongoing medical management is a cornerstone of long-term care for POTS. This typically involves a regimen of medications to manage the heart rate, blood pressure, and blood volume, all of which are key in minimizing symptoms. However, the effectiveness of these medications can change over time, and regular follow-ups with healthcare professionals are essential to monitor the condition and adjust treatments accordingly. Keeping a detailed symptom diary can be incredibly useful in these appointments, as it provides a clear picture of how various factors affect the individual's condition.

Lifestyle adjustments play a crucial role in managing POTS. Diet is a significant aspect, with many individuals benefiting from increased salt and fluid intake to enhance blood volume. Small, frequent meals can also help prevent significant shifts in blood pressure and heart rate associated with larger meals. An exercise regimen tailored to the individual's tolerance level is important. Starting with low-impact exercises and gradually increasing the intensity can help improve cardiovascular fitness and reduce symptoms. Good sleep hygiene is essential for managing fatigue, a common symptom of POTS. This includes maintaining a regular sleep schedule, creating a comfortable sleep environment, and addressing any sleep disorders.

Addressing the psychological impact of POTS is equally important. Chronic illnesses can take a toll on mental health, leading to increased stress, anxiety, and depression. Regular consultations with mental health professionals, engaging in stress-reduction techniques like mindfulness and relaxation exercises, and participating in cognitive-behavioral therapy can provide significant mental health benefits. Support groups and online forums offer platforms to connect with others who understand the challenges of living with POTS, providing emotional support and practical advice.

Future planning and goal setting are important for individuals with POTS. This might involve making adjustments in career plans, seeking accommodations in educational settings, or finding flexible work arrangements that consider the fluctuating nature of POTS. Setting realistic and flexible goals helps in maintaining a sense of control and direction in life.

Building a strong support network is vital. This network should include healthcare providers knowledgeable about POTS, as well as family, friends, and peers who understand the condition. Engaging in patient advocacy and community education initiatives can empower individuals and help increase public awareness and understanding of POTS.

In conclusion, long-term management of POTS is a dynamic process that involves a combination of medical treatment, lifestyle adjustments, psychological support, and community engagement. It requires an adaptable approach, informed by ongoing education about the condition, and supported by a network of healthcare professionals, family, and peers. With the right strategies and support, individuals with POTS can manage their symptoms effectively and maintain a fulfilling and active life.

CHAPTER FIVE: THE FUTURE OF POTS TREATMENT AND RESEARCH

This chapter, "The Future of POTS Treatment and Research," delves into the evolving landscape of Postural Orthostatic Tachycardia Syndrome (POTS) care and scientific exploration. It presents the latest advancements and significant research findings in the treatment of POTS, highlighting the progress and emerging therapies that offer hope to those affected. The chapter also explores the increasing role of technology in managing POTS, from innovative diagnostic tools to novel treatment approaches, illustrating how technology is transforming patient care.

Additionally, it provides insights into the realm of clinical trials, guiding POTS patients on how to participate and what to expect from these vital research endeavors. Looking ahead, the chapter envisions the future possibilities and advancements in the understanding and treatment of POTS, painting an optimistic picture of continued progress and enhanced patient outcomes.

Current Research and Emerging Treatments

The field of Postural Orthostatic Tachycardia Syndrome (POTS) research and treatment is rapidly evolving, marked by significant advancements in understanding and managing this complex condition. The current landscape of POTS research is multifaceted, encompassing various areas from deepening our understanding of its pathophysiology to exploring innovative treatment options.

In terms of understanding the condition, recent research efforts are increasingly focused on unraveling the intricate pathophysiology of POTS. This includes studying the dysfunction of the autonomic nervous system, which plays a crucial role in the condition, and examining factors related to blood volume regulation and heart rate control. Researchers are delving into the potential genetic basis of POTS, exploring whether genetic markers or predispositions contribute to its development. Such research is pivotal as it could lead to more personalized and effective treatment approaches in the future.

Pharmacological advancements constitute a significant area of development in POTS treatment. The development and testing of new medications specifically targeting the underlying mechanisms of POTS are ongoing. These medications aim to stabilize heart rate, improve blood volume regulation, and alleviate other symptoms associated with autonomic dysfunction. Clinical trials are critical in this context as they help determine the efficacy and safety of these new pharmacological treatments, ultimately guiding the development of effective medication regimens for individuals with POTS.

Non-pharmacological treatments are also an important aspect of POTS management. Research continues to support the effectiveness of lifestyle interventions, such as dietary modifications, which often include increased salt and fluid intake to enhance blood volume. Physical therapy and structured exercise programs are also emphasized, as they can improve cardiovascular conditioning and reduce symptoms over time. Additionally, therapies like biofeedback, acupuncture, and other complementary treatments are being explored for their potential benefits in symptom management, offering alternative or supplementary options to conventional medical treatments.

The role of technology in managing POTS is another area of significant advancement. Wearable technology that monitors vital signs like heart rate and blood pressure is becoming increasingly integral to daily management for many individuals with POTS. These devices offer real-time data that can be crucial for understanding and managing the condition. Advances in telemedicine are also proving beneficial, especially in improving access to specialized care for POTS patients, enabling remote consultations and monitoring, which is particularly valuable for those with mobility challenges or living in remote areas.

Collaborative research efforts, both nationally and internationally, are enhancing the pace and breadth of discoveries in the field of POTS. This collaboration is not only between researchers but also includes engagement with POTS patients and advocacy groups. Such involvement ensures that research efforts are aligned with the actual needs and experiences of those living with the condition, making them more relevant and impactful.

Looking ahead, the future of POTS research and treatment seems to be heading towards the realm of precision medicine. This approach promises more personalized treatment strategies, tailored to the individual characteristics of each patient, and integrates pharmacological, lifestyle, and technological interventions. Such a comprehensive approach is expected to significantly improve the quality of life for individuals with POTS.

In conclusion, the current and future landscape of POTS treatment and research is characterized by a dynamic and integrated approach that combines medical advancements, lifestyle modifications, technological innovations, and patient-centered research. This holistic approach is essential for developing more effective and personalized management strategies for POTS, ultimately enhancing patient care and outcomes.

The Role of Technology in Managing POTS

The integration of technology in the management of Postural Orthostatic Tachycardia Syndrome (POTS) marks a significant advancement in how this condition is understood and managed. The application of innovative technological solutions is profoundly influencing patient care, from diagnosis to daily symptom management.

Wearable technology has become an essential tool for individuals with POTS. Advanced smartwatches and fitness trackers, equipped with sensors to monitor heart rate and blood pressure, offer a way for patients to keep track of these vital signs continuously. This real-time monitoring is invaluable for POTS, where symptoms can change rapidly and unpredictably. Patients can observe how various activities, stressors, or environmental conditions affect their symptoms, enabling them to make informed decisions about managing their daily activities and lifestyles.

Mobile health applications are enhancing the way individuals manage POTS. These apps allow for detailed symptom tracking, medication management, and even dietary logging. For instance, patients can record episodes of dizziness, monitor fluctuations in heart rate, and note correlations with specific activities or foods.

This level of detailed health logging is incredibly useful during medical appointments, providing a comprehensive view of the patient's health over time and aiding in the effectiveness of treatment strategies.

Telemedicine has emerged as a vital resource, particularly beneficial for POTS patients who may face challenges with physical mobility. It facilitates regular access to healthcare providers through virtual consultations, allowing for consistent medical oversight without the need for physical travel. Additionally, telemedicine opens up access to specialized care, enabling patients to consult with POTS experts who may not be available locally.

Technological advancements in diagnostic equipment have significantly improved the accuracy and efficiency of diagnosing POTS. Innovations in tilt table testing and non-invasive hemodynamic monitoring are providing clinicians with more comprehensive data. Furthermore, therapies such as biofeedback and neurofeedback, which use technology to help patients gain control over certain bodily functions like heart rate, are being explored for their potential benefits in symptom management.

The role of technology extends into the realm of research, where big data analytics and artificial intelligence are making strides in POTS research. These technologies are being used to analyze large datasets to identify patterns, and potential triggers, and understand the broader impacts of POTS. This analysis can help in identifying biomarkers and predicting treatment responses, contributing to the development of more targeted and effective treatment strategies.

Looking ahead, advancements in wearable technology promise even more sophisticated monitoring capabilities, potentially offering deeper insights into the autonomic changes associated with POTS. The future also holds the potential for an integrated health management system that combines wearables, mobile health apps, and telemedicine. Such a system could provide real-time, personalized recommendations for managing POTS, revolutionizing the daily management of the condition.

In summary, technology is playing an increasingly crucial role in the management of POTS, offering new ways to monitor symptoms, manage health, and receive medical care. These technological advancements are not only improving the quality of life for individuals with POTS but are also opening up new avenues for research and understanding of this complex condition. As technology continues to advance, it holds great promise for further enhancing patient care and treatment outcomes for those living with POTS.

Participating in Clinical Trials

Participating in clinical trials is an invaluable way for individuals with Postural Orthostatic Tachycardia Syndrome (POTS) to contribute to the advancement of medical research and potentially access new treatments. The journey from finding appropriate trials to understanding the intricacies of participation is crucial for individuals considering this path.

Finding suitable clinical trials for POTS involves thorough research. Databases like ClinicalTrials.gov provide detailed listings of ongoing and upcoming studies worldwide. Here, individuals can search for trials specific to POTS, filtering them based on location, eligibility criteria, and study status. Beyond online databases, healthcare providers, particularly those specializing in POTS or related fields, can be invaluable resources in identifying relevant clinical trials. They can offer guidance on suitable options based on a patient's medical history and current health status.

Once a potentially suitable trial is identified, the next step is understanding and meeting the eligibility criteria. These criteria, which can include specific medical history, symptom severity, age, and overall health, are designed to ensure participant safety and the study's validity. The enrollment process often includes initial screenings, such as medical questionnaires, physical examinations, and thorough reviews of medical history, to ensure that potential participants meet all the study's requirements.

Participants in clinical trials can expect to receive a comprehensive overview of the study protocol. This overview includes the purpose of the research, details about the treatment or intervention being tested, the duration of the trial, and the schedule of tests and assessments. Participants are required to sign an informed consent form, which outlines the potential risks, benefits, rights, and responsibilities associated with the trial. It is vital to read this document carefully and ask the research team any clarifying questions.

Clinical trials do involve certain risks, such as unknown side effects from experimental treatments. However, they also offer potential benefits, including access to new treatments and contributing to research that may improve POTS management and understanding in the future. During the trial, participants will undergo regular health assessments to monitor their response to the treatment and identify any side effects, ensuring participant safety and the integrity of the study's results.

After the conclusion of a trial, most studies include follow-up care to monitor participants' health and manage any long-term effects of the treatment. Participants often receive updates about the overall findings of the study, providing insights into the efficacy and safety of the treatment.

Deciding to participate in a clinical trial is a significant decision that should be made after careful consideration and discussion with healthcare providers, family, and the research team. For individuals with POTS, involvement in clinical trials is not only an opportunity for potential personal health benefits but also a meaningful way to contribute to the broader understanding and treatment of this challenging condition.

The Horizon of POTS Care

The future of Postural Orthostatic Tachycardia Syndrome (POTS) care is on the cusp of significant advancements, with promising research and technological developments shaping a more hopeful landscape for those affected by this condition. This future is characterized by a deeper understanding of the disorder, personalized treatment approaches, and improved quality of life for patients.

In the realm of understanding POTS, ongoing research is vital. Efforts are being made to unravel the complexities of the autonomic nervous system's involvement in POTS and to delineate its various subtypes, each potentially requiring different treatment approaches. The investigation into genetic factors and underlying mechanisms is crucial, as it paves the way for treatments that target the root causes of the condition rather than just managing symptoms.

Personalized medicine stands at the forefront of future POTS care. The goal is to tailor treatments to each individual's unique set of symptoms, genetic makeup, and treatment responses. This approach promises more effective and efficient management of the condition, moving away from the traditional one-size-fits-all strategy. Personalized treatment plans could include specific medications, lifestyle modifications, and other therapies, all finely tuned to the patient's needs.

Technological innovations are expected to play a transformative role in managing POTS. Wearable technology is anticipated to become more advanced, providing detailed and accurate monitoring of critical physiological parameters such as blood volume, heart rate variability, and more. These devices will offer real-time insights into how different activities and environmental factors affect patients, leading to more informed daily management. Additionally, the expansion of telemedicine will enhance access to specialized care, making it easier for patients to receive consistent, expert guidance without the need for extensive travel.

The development of improved diagnostic tools and criteria is another critical area of focus for the future. Enhanced diagnostic methods will facilitate earlier and more accurate diagnoses of POTS, improving the chances of effective treatment. This includes advancements in tilt table testing, greater recognition and understanding of POTS among healthcare professionals, and the development of biomarkers for more straightforward identification of the syndrome.

Expanding treatment options for POTS is a key aspect of future care. Researchers are exploring new pharmacological treatments specifically designed to address the underlying dysfunctions in POTS. Additionally, novel therapies such as immunotherapy and stem cell therapy are under investigation, offering hope for more definitive and long-lasting solutions to the symptoms of POTS.

Collaboration and awareness are pivotal for the future of POTS care. Increased collaboration between researchers, clinicians, and patients will drive forward advancements in treatment and understanding. Greater awareness of POTS, both within the medical community and the general public, is essential for ensuring timely diagnoses, appropriate treatment, and adequate support for those living with the condition.

Lastly, the focus on improving the overall quality of life for POTS patients is gaining prominence. Future care strategies will likely emphasize not only physical symptom management but also support for the mental and emotional challenges associated with living with a chronic illness. A more holistic approach to care, integrating physical, psychological, and social support, will become increasingly important in managing POTS.

In summary, the horizon of POTS care is bright with the potential for enhanced understanding, individualized treatment approaches, and improved patient outcomes. As research progresses and technology advances, the future holds significant promise for those affected by Postural Orthostatic Tachycardia Syndrome, offering hope for a better quality of life and more effective management of the condition.

CONCLUSION

As we conclude this comprehensive exploration of Postural Orthostatic Tachycardia Syndrome (POTS), it's important to reflect on the key takeaways and empower you, the reader, for the journey ahead. This book aims to provide a thorough understanding of POTS, delving into its symptoms, diagnosis, management strategies, and the latest research developments. We've explored how technology is reshaping the landscape of POTS care and the importance of personal advocacy and continued learning in managing this condition.

The journey with POTS is unique for each individual, marked by its challenges and triumphs. We hope that the insights shared here have equipped you with the knowledge and tools to take an active role in managing your condition. Remember, you are the most important advocate for your health, and staying informed and proactive is key to navigating the complexities of POTS. Embrace the support systems available to you, whether they be healthcare professionals, support groups, online communities, or family and friends. Their support, combined with your resilience and determination, will be invaluable assets on this journey.

We encourage you to continue the conversation about POTS beyond the pages of this book. Engage in ongoing learning, participate in community advocacy, and contribute to raising awareness about this condition. Your experiences and insights are powerful tools in the collective effort to enhance understanding and treatment of POTS.

Finally, we end this book with a message of encouragement and hope. While living with POTS can be challenging, there are continuously evolving treatments and a growing community of support. The future holds promise for improved care and a deeper understanding of POTS. Let this book be a starting point for your journey, a companion along the way, and a reminder that you are not alone in this. With determination, support, and continued advancements in POTS care, there is every reason to be hopeful for a brighter and healthier future.